My Silence is Broken

For the survivors of

www.thehuntinggroundfilm.com (2015)

www.spotlight.com (2015)

And

Everyone else who has not spoken yet

My Silence is Broken

A Workbook for Helping Survivors

Of Sexual Abuse and Rape

It was not your fault

Gary Sellors

Published in 2015 by Amazon

Copyright © Gary Sellors 2015

ISBN: 978-1-51865-159-5

This is for my Mum, Dad and my rescue cat Tommy

Acknowledgements

I wish to say a huge thank you to all the people who have shared their personal stories in this book and all those that did not make this final version.

To those of you who shared your stories. By having the courage to do so, you will have inspired many people who haven't told anyone yet.

Words cannot convey just how important a gift this is. Thank you again.

I would like to thank Emmy Fisher, who helped start this project in so many ways. I'd like to thank my very special friend Cathie Furlong, for making some important suggestions.

A good mention to the Police Forces and Probation trusts that I have shared my knowledge and experience with. Thank you to the social media comments I have received in moving this project to its final stage.

The many people who have supported and encouraged me, including Helen and Anna.

Especially those friends who are doctors, healers and therapists, with whom I have had so many stimulating conversations about health and medicine, and who have reassured me that my 'crazy' ideas do make intuitive and scientific sense.

I'm just so happy that I can inspire, motivate and help people to grow in confidence. From all the cases that I have worked with, they have really trusted me, in telling me their traumatic stories. Every story has been an emotional journey.

Thank you

Gary Sellors September 2015

My Silence is Broken

This is a workbook for survivors of sexual abuse and rape, who may want to seek help but be unsure who to speak to or where to go.

It is very common for survivors of sexual abuse not to report their experience.

This work book is for anyone looking for advice and support in taking the first step of speaking about their experience and seeking help.

No one needs to know that they are completing this work book. It is designed to be completed on their own.

Please remember if you are being abused or are in danger, always call 999 (UK) immediately.

Trigger Warning:

This workbook contains information and real-life stories which may be distressing. If at any time during this workbook, you become distressed or feel that you may harm yourself or others, please seek help immediately from an appropriate organisation using the contact details provided in this book.

Welcome to the My Silence is Broken Workbook

This workbook has been designed to help and support people who have been affected by sexual abuse or rape. In 2015, media attention to historic cases has brought forward so many stories from people who are now speaking out and saying that they were sexually abused or raped in the past.

The BBC News reported in June 2015 that there is not enough intervention work being done towards helping people affected. This work book is a step that survivors can take on their own, in their own time, which will empower them to seek appropriate help and support.

There are many reasons why survivors may not report sexual violence, including feelings of shame and fear that they will not be believed. Some attitudes of the police force and courts towards survivors of rape and sexual abuse have historically been negative, which has damaged trust in the systems set up to support victims of sexual violence.

These factors can make it very difficult for people to feel that they will be, or have been, listened to.

This programme works because unlike other support projects, it can be completed in a person's own time and private space. This is the most important aspect of this workbook.

Many survivors feel unable to tell anyone about their experiences of sexual abuse and rape, and therefore this book can help to prepare and empower them to seek help and tell their story.

This workbook is designed to help people:

- Grow in confidence in preparing to talk to someone about their experience of sexual abuse and rape

- Allow time and space to reflect on and understand what has happened

- Validate their feelings about their experiences

- Access appropriate help and support

Who is Gary Sellors?

Gary has been providing specialist therapeutic interventions for people affected by sexual violence and rape for over 18 years.

His background includes working with Hertfordshire and Sussex Police forces for 4 years as a Police Special Constable, over 5 years with Sussex and Surrey, BENCH and NPS Probation Trusts working directly with sex offenders on their release.

Gary is a qualified Doctor of Clinical Hypnotherapy and an intuitive healer, incorporating his extensive therapeutic knowledge with his practical experience in working with survivors of rape and sexual violence, to support them in moving forwards in their lives.

Gary is a fellowship member of the London College of Clinical Hypnosis and a follows the guidelines of National Institute for Health and Care Excellence (N.I.C.E).

Real life stories 1

My client was abused from the age of 10 years, by the baby sitter. He would come around once a week, as her parents would like to go out once a week.

The baby sitter would kindly look after her and her younger sister aged 6. The parents thought at the time it was lovely as he was a nice man and never wanted any money for babysitting.

She remembers, him coming in to her bedroom, and saying what he wanted her to do and that if she didn't do what he wanted, he said he would go and play with her younger sister. She had no choice to do what he wanted to protect her sister. This carried on for over 4 years.

She recalls being taken to a special doctor, by the baby sitter, who gave her tablets to ensure that she didn't get pregnant. The doctor would always give her a very close examination as well and take photos.

The perpetrator got caught in the end outside a school. He was put away for 7 years. The doctor went abroad.

Helpful Contact Numbers

Greater London Organisations:

The Havens, St. Mary's Hospital, Paddington, London
- http://www.thehavens.org.uk/
- 0207 886 1101 (9am – 5pm) 0207 886 6666 (all other times)

One In Four (London SE6)
- http://www.oneinfour.org.uk/
- 020 8697 2112

Women and Girls Network (West London)
- http://www.wgn.org.uk/
- National helpline: 020 7610 4345

National Organisations:

Rape Crisis
- http://rapecrisis.org.uk/
- National helpline: 0808 802 9999

The Samaritans
- http://www.samaritans.org/
- National helpline: 08457 90 90 90

Women's Aid / Refuge
- http://www.womensaid.org.uk/
- National helpline: 0808 2000 247

NAPAC National Association for People Abused in Childhood
- www.napac.org.uk
- National helpline: 0800 085 3330

Mankind UK
- http://www.mankindcounselling.org.uk
- 01273 510 447

SURVIVORS UK
- https://www.survivorsuk.org/
- National Helpline: 0845 221 201 / 0208 691 8236

About Sexual Violence, Abuse and Rape

Before we begin the work book, the following section will help to provide more information about sexual violence and rape, and hopefully dispel some common myths. Sexual violence is not often spoken about by the media or within our communities, and so a lot of misinformation can spread.

Below are some frequently asked questions about sexual violence, abuse and rape.

What is sexual violence?

Sexual violence is defined as "any unwanted sexual act or activity" (Rape Crisis, 2015)

There are many different types of sexual violence, including rape, sexual assault, sexual harassment, child sexual abuse, rape within relationships, sexual exploitation or trafficking, forced marriage, female genital mutilation and others.

In this workbook, the terms sexual violence and rape are used to refer to any unwanted sexual activity.

Sexual violence can affect anyone, regardless of gender, sexual orientation, culture or other factors. It can be perpetrated by a stranger, or someone known to the person, such as a partner, ex-partner, friend, family member, colleague or acquaintance.

If you have been, or are experiencing, sexual violence, it's not your fault and you're not alone.

Is it my fault I experienced sexual abuse?

No. It isn't your fault if you have experienced sexual abuse or rape. People who sexually abuse others often make the people they abuse feel guilty and ashamed about what happened.

This is so that they keep quiet about it. Sexual abuse can make you feel confused and scared. Even if they say it is your fault, it is never your fault. They are responsible for what they have done to you.

You have done nothing wrong.

Can men experience sexual abuse?

Men can also experience sexual abuse and rape, both from women and other men of all sexual orientations. This is just as difficult and traumatising for men as it is for women, yet some men find that the people around them are less understanding or that there is less support for them.

The majority of male rape is perpetrated by heterosexual men on other heterosexual men. For the male rape survivor, this can cause them to have anxieties about their sexuality. It is very common for men to have had an erection during or after the assault.

This is purely physical reaction, a response to fear and adrenalin, and does not mean you enjoyed it or deserved to be raped. Some straight men might wonder if being raped means they are gay, or that they were raped because they are gay. However rape is not about sexual gratification or sexuality, it is an act of control and humiliation. It does not have any bearing on the sexual orientation of the victim.

What is sexual abuse in childhood?

It is beginning to be acknowledged that childhood sexual abuse happens a lot more frequently than most people have believed, or wanted to believe.

Childhood sexual abuse could include the following.

- Being cuddled or kissed in a way that left the survivor feeling uncomfortable.
- Having their breasts or genitals touched.
- Being bathed in a way that felt uncomfortable.
- Being forced to perform oral sex, or having it performed on them.
- Having their vagina or anus penetrated by a penis, finger or object.
- Having to pose for photographs or being videoed having sex.

Sexual exploitation is a form of sexual abuse, in which a young person is manipulated or forced into taking part in a sexual act.

 This could be as part of a relationship which seems to be normal and loving or in return for attention, affection, money, drugs, alcohol or somewhere to stay.

What is grooming?

In many cases of sexual abuse in childhood, survivors will have been "groomed" by an abusing adult, who befriends them and makes them feel special by buying them gifts or giving them lots of attention. Usually the abuser will have power of some kind over the young person.

It may be that they are older or more emotionally mature, physically stronger, or that they are in a position where they are able to control the young person.

Grooming is a word used to describe how people who want to sexually harm children and young people get close to them, and often their families, and gain their trust.

Grooming in the real world can take place in all kinds of places – in the home or local neighbourhood, the child's school, youth and sports clubs or the church.

Online grooming may occur by people forming relationships with children and pretending to be their friend.

They do this by finding out information about their potential victim and trying to establish the likelihood of the child telling.

Can sexual abuse occur in relationships?

Sexual abuse is most often perpetrated by someone close to the survivor, including spouses, romantic or sexual partners.

There are many terms for sexual abuse in a relationship, including intimate partner sexual violence, intimate partner rape, marital rape, spousal rape and domestic violence.

Regardless of the status of a relationship, it is never okay for someone to engage in a sexual activity without the other person's consent.

Often when there is sexual abuse in a relationship, other kinds of abuse, such as emotional, psychological or physical abuse, may also occur.

It may be very challenging for someone in a relationship with a perpetrator of sexual abuse to come forward for many reasons.

They may not realise that the abuse constitutes sexual assault, be scared for their safety or the safety of children, or still have strong feelings for the abuser.

What do people typically experience following sexual abuse?

Following a traumatic event, everyone reacts differently and there is no right or wrong way to respond. Whatever you are feeling is completely valid. There are some common thoughts, feelings and responses to sexual abuse. Some people might experience a lot of them, and some none at all. They include:

- Being in shock if the attack happened recently. You may feel numb or unemotional, start shaking, crying or laughing, or be physically sick.
- You may feel unclean or dirty, even after washing.
- Feeling guilty, ashamed or responsible for the abuse.
- Experiencing flashbacks or reliving the event, having nightmares or intrusive thoughts. You may have difficulty sleeping.
- Feeling scared, lonely, vulnerable or anxious.
- Finding it difficult to be alone or go out by yourself.
- Having little confidence in yourself and trust in others.
- Feeling worthless, hating yourself, feeling suicidal or wanting to harm yourself.
- Finding it difficult to cope with day to day life.
- Experiencing difficulties with sex or in relationships.

For more information about sexual abuse and rape, please refer to the organisations provided on the useful contacts page.

"A hero is an ordinary individual who finds the strength to persevere and endure in spite of overwhelming obstacles" ~ Christopher Reeve

Real life stories 2

"I was abused by my father, from the age of 13. It started when my mum started working in the evenings as we didn't have enough money coming in.

He made me not tell anyone or he would hurt the family cat that we had. He left me alone at 15. I didn't know what to do, and did at the time become promiscuous and got a name for myself".

Now age 47.

Workbook Sections

1. Tell your story

2. Understanding blame

3. Acceptance and letting go

4. Coping with guilt and shame

5. Removing the movie

6. Time to relax

7. Deciding who to tell or 'if' to tell?

8. The future you

9. Suggested reading

Section One: Tell your story

The importance of stories

Stories are how we understand the world around us, and place our experiences into the context of our life.

We understand our past experiences through stories. We tell stories to relate to other people, to share ideas and experiences, to explain what has happened or is happening to us.

For survivors of sexual abuse, telling the story of their experience can be extremely difficult. At their core, rape and sexual violence are not sexual acts, but crimes of control. People do not abuse others for sexual gratification, but to intimidate, humiliate and silence their victim.

Many survivors feel that they have no voice, that their story will not be believed, or that they are unable to speak about their experience. Some people may have been silenced directly by the perpetrator of the violence, through threats or their position.

When we experience traumas such as sexual abuse, especially when we feel silenced, the mind tries to protect itself by trying to block out the memory of the experience. This can result in flashbacks, distress and difficult emotions including fear, anxiety, shame, anger and despair.

Putting a traumatic event into words can be incredibly difficult, upsetting and painful as memories and thoughts are relived. You may have shut thoughts or feelings away in a box which has remained unopened for some time. But the act of silencing a person's story, whether this silencing is enforced by the perpetrator or happens internally by the survivor, can make it more difficult to heal and let go of the memories and emotions.

This exercise guides you to put your own story into words. It is the beginning of finding your voice and breaking the silence around your experiences; not to tell anyone else initially, but to know and understand your story for yourself.

ALL rape is about humiliation, power and control.

Rape is NOT about sex

About the exercise:

The simple, effective technique has been used for many successful therapeutic interventions. It works in the case of sexual abuse and rape because it can help to open a door into your experience, to approach memories, thoughts and feelings in total safety and privacy.

Please remember that this is an exercise that you complete on your own. Allow 20 minutes to do it, use this page and have a lot of blank spare pages to write on and a nice flowing pen. Please don't worry about spelling, neatness, grammar or how it ends up looking - no one is going to see it. It doesn't need to make sense, or be accurate, or go into every detail – just write whatever comes up that is meaningful for you.

There are two key things that make this exercise work very well. Firstly, no one will read this work, as you destroy it straight afterwards, so you can write absolutely anything and everything. It is really important that you trust this exercise.

The other key thing is that you MUST NOT read what you have written, as what you have written down will have temporarily left your mind and it is now on the paper in front of you. This is an exercise in letting go, so there is no need to check your work or read it back.

"So often survivors have had their experiences denied, trivialized, or distorted. Writing is an important avenue for healing because it gives you an opportunity to define your own reality. You can say: This did happen to me. It was bad. It was the fault & responsibility of the adult. I was - and am – innocent"

~ Ellen Bass

Real life stories 3

"I was 9 at the time and used to play games with my brothers best mate, who I thought was cool and a little older than me. He was 15.

We used to play in the woods and in our parents garden, we had a lot of fun. One day, he asked if I wanted to play a game called blindfold where I had to guess what he would put in my mouth. I said don't put a spider in there please".

After a few normal items including vegetables, he then undid his trousers and put his penis in my mouth, it took me a few seconds to realise what he was doing.

I started crying, and he quickly did his trousers up and told me not to tell anyone, as it was just a game. It took me 7 years to tell someone.

My brother's best mate was put on the sex offender register list for 10 years. He lost his job".

"I'm not going to tell you to get over it. I'm going to help you get through it"

~ anon

How to complete this exercise:

Write down every single thought, feeling, resentment or frustration relating to your experience, no matter how hurtful, sexual, harmful or difficult.

Don't focus on how it looks or what you have written; just keep writing for twenty minutes. It may be difficult to start, but persevere and write down anything that comes to mind.

Write for 20 minutes, and then stop. It is now time to destroy it. Some people like to set it alight and watch it burn, others have placed it in water to drown it or dug a hole in the garden and buried it; do whatever feels right for you.

Please remember: don't read it, show no one and destroy it afterwards.

Then on day 2, repeat same exercise, with the blank paper and pen again.

Start by writing what you remember from yesterday; you won't remember everything you wrote, and some new thoughts and feelings will come up.

Only write for 20 minutes then destroy again.

Please don't show any one and do not read it yourself. (This is really important, if you were to reread it, all those thoughts, feelings go back in your mind again).

On day 3, repeat the same exercise, with blank sheets and a nice pen. Again, try to remember what you wrote on day 2, adding any new thoughts or feelings.

At this point, you may find that it is more difficult to recall what you have written, which is why this exercise works so well.

By day 4, you may start to wonder what you are going to write for 20 minutes, as by now you will have started to clear some space in your mind.

Always destroy your work afterwards; this part for a lot of people can be very rewarding.

Some people have a ceremony, for letting go.

You may like to light a candle or incense, meditate or do some deep breathing, as you let go of the thoughts and feelings written on the paper.

This is a very trusted and effective exercise. Release and be free.

Day 1

(Please have additional paper available, or tear this page out)

Tell your story - what happened to you?

Day 2

(Please have additional paper available, or tear this page out)

Tell your story - what happened to you?

Day 3

(Please have additional paper available, or tear this page out)

Tell your story - what happened to you?

Day 4

(Please have additional paper available, or tear this page out)

Tell your story - what happened to you?

Real life stories 4

"I was at a mates party on a Saturday night. I was 18 at the time, I'm now 39. My girlfriends at the time did like to drink a bit too much.

I woke up at the party to find myself lying on the kitchen table in the middle of the kitchen, with no knickers on, my legs in the air and a complete stranger, having sex with me, as I could feel him inside of me.

What made it worse was his mates were filming him having sex with me.

I was ashamed of myself and my friends disowned me, as how could I let one of my girlfriend's boyfriend's do that to me.

He said that I made him do that to me. It took many years to come to terms with what happened and get away from everyone who had seen the video footage.

I tried to kill myself 3 times. I am married with 2 lovely children now, BUT, my husband doesn't know what happened".

Section Two: Understanding Blame

You are not to blame.

Many survivors of sexual abuse feel that they are in some way responsible or to blame for the attack. Some survivors may feel, or have felt, ashamed, dirty, humiliated or guilty about their experiences. These feelings are a very common response to the helplessness and powerlessness experienced during sexual violence.

Misconceptions about rape and sexual abuse, often portrayed in the media, may also affect the way we perceive what has happened to us.

This may lead to feelings of self-doubt, self-blame or confusion about whether rape or sexual violence has occurred.

In every case of sexual abuse and rape, the perpetrator carries 100% of the responsibility, and 100% of the blame.

- What you were wearing does not matter
- What you were doing at the time does not matter
- Where you were and what time it was does not matter
- Whether you were already in a relationship with the perpetrator does not matter
- Whether you had taken alcohol or drugs does not matter
- Whether you consented to sex then changed your mind does not matter
- Your past experiences and sexual history does not matter
- Whether you were forced to participate in sexual acts does not matter
- Whether you struggled, called out or resisted or not, does not matter

Sexual abuse is always the fault of the perpetrator. There are no circumstances where it is ever justified for a person to rape or sexually assault another person.

There are no circumstances where a person who commits a sexual act or activity without the person's consent, does not constitute sexual violence.

About the exercise:

Although you may understand at a logical level that the perpetrator is entirely to blame for the sexual abuse you have experienced, healing cannot take place until you feel it deep down.

This involves letting go of self-doubt and self-blame, gaining some closure on any thoughts you may have had about being in any way responsible for the attack.

By looking deeply at who you have been blaming and why, then re-evaluating your answers, you may find that thoughts, whether conscious or unconscious, come to the surface which need to be addressed and put into the context of your story.

How to complete the exercise:

Below are two columns: who do you blame, and why do you blame them. Start by listing who you blame, then as you do, write down any thoughts or feelings that come up connected to each person.

It does not need to make sense, and you may find that new thoughts or feelings come up which you have not noticed before. That's ok; just note them down without judging yourself for them.

Who	Why
Who	**Why**
Who	**Why**
Who	**Why**
Who	**Why**

As you reflect on your answers, you may start to get a deeper understanding of who you have been blaming for your experience.

When you look at the 'who' answers now, ask yourself:

- Is the answer really true? YES / NO
- Was I responsible for what happened? YES / NO
- Did I really deserve it? YES / NO
- Did I attract it? YES / NO
- Could I have done something differently? YES/ NO

On reflection of these answers, you might start to notice a shift in your thinking about how responsible each person was in the situation.

What is often learnt from this exercise is that the balance of blame starts to shift from you as the survivor and on to the perpetrator, where it should stay.

After reflection, who do you blame now?

If this answer has changed, why and how has it changed?

"Nothing in the universe can stop you from letting go and starting over." ~ Guy Finley

Keep your children safe online

Teach your children the five key Childnet SMART rules which remind young people to be SMART online. You should go through these tips with your children.

S – SAFE. Keep safe by being careful not to give out personal information – such as your name, email, phone number, home address, or school name – to people who you don't know online.

M – MEETING. Meeting someone you have only been in touch with online can be dangerous. Only do so with your parents'/carers' permissions & when they can be present.

A – ACCEPTING. Accepting e-mails, IM messages or opening files from people you don't know or trust can be dangerous – they may contain viruses or nasty messages.

R – RELIABLE. Someone online may be lying about who they are, and information you find on the internet may not be reliable.

T – TELL. Your parent, carer or a trusted adult if someone or something makes you feel uncomfortable or worried.

If you want to ask a question or talk through any issues or concerns, call the **Stop it Now!** Confidential, Free phone helpline on 0808 1000 900. (UK)

The helpline is available from 9am-9pm Monday to Thursday and 9am-5pm Fridays.

Alternatively you can contact us for help and advice via email at this address: help@stopitnow.org.uk, with a response in 48 hours.

More information available from Parentsprotect.co.uk

Section Three: Acceptance and Letting Go

Why is acceptance important?

One of the mind's defences against traumatic events is denial. You may have found yourself 'blocking out' thoughts about your experience of sexual violence, or justifying what has happened. Pushing away the pain, fear or trauma can make emotional wounds worse in the long term.

It can take a long time to come to terms with the idea of that you have experienced sexual abuse or rape. In some cases, the process of acceptance can take many years.

Perpetrators commit sexual abuse because they want to control and harm others. Acceptance helps to take back this control. It is about standing up and saying 'yes you hurt me, but I am stronger than this and I will get through it'.

Acceptance is **not** about forgiving the perpetrator for what they have done, or being passive. It is about acknowledging that we cannot change events in our past, but by accepting them we can move forwards, let go, and start to heal.

"Acceptance does not excuse their behaviour. Acceptance prevents their behaviour from destroying your heart."

What does it mean to let go?

The impact of rape and sexual abuse goes far beyond the immediate consequences. Emotions such as fear, guilt, anxiety, shame, anger, helplessness and despair can have long-lasting effects which can hold us back from living the life that we want to live.

Letting go is important because the perpetrator is taking up rent-free space your mind which they do not deserve. You have many more interesting, beautiful and loving thoughts to occupy your mind, so much potential to create a life you love.

Although you may not ever forget, or totally come to terms with, your experience of sexual abuse, like any trauma it is possible to recover and create a meaningful, happy life by healing. It is possible to be free of the emotions holding you back, by gradually letting them go.

About the exercise:

This letter may be the hardest thing you will ever write. Please remember that no one will ever know that you have written it, you will never post it, and no one will ever read it apart from yourself.

The point of writing the letter is for YOU. You are now just starting to regain the control back in your life. This is proving you are now starting to let go of any feelings of pain, fear, helplessness, shame or trauma. It is a long process, but this may be the first step.

This letter is about acknowledging that there is a future and that you are free to create it. Letting go is a long and difficult process, but it is the path to emotional freedom.

"The truth is, unless you let go, unless you forgive yourself, unless you forgive the situation, unless you realize that the situation is over, you cannot move forward"

~ Steve Maraboli

Real life stories 6

I'm now 27 years old and been in a relationship with my boyfriend for the last 3 years. I'm still unable to have a full physical sexually relationship with my boyfriend, which he understands and supports me, although I feel bad that I am not pleasing him.

I was sexually abused by my step dad at 11 and at 19 I was drugged on a night out and raped, by a guy I had just met.

How to complete the exercise:

Complete the following phrases, using extra paper as needed.

I accept that you…

I accept that you wanted to control and hurt me, but I am taking back control because…

Note: Sometimes the abuser may not have the mental awareness of what they were doing?

I am letting go of…

I accept that awful things do happen in life and that I cannot change the past. I am now beginning to restore my life. I have so much to look forward to, such as…

It's important to make a decision that you are going to move on. It won't happen automatically. You will have to stand up and say:

"I don't care how hard this is, I don't care how scared / angry / hopeless / anxious / ashamed I feel. I am not going to let this get the better of me. I am now moving on with my life."

You may like to try repeating this as an affirmation, using words that feel right for you.

Section Four – Coping with Guilt and Shame

Why do I feel ashamed and guilty?

It is extremely common for survivors of sexual abuse or rape to feel guilty and/or ashamed. Sexual abuse is not an act of passion or lust, but an attempt to control and humiliate. The perpetrator evokes feelings of guilt and shame in the person they are attacking, in order to keep them scared and silent.

There is no case in which the victim of sexual abuse or rape is in any way responsible for the actions of the perpetrator. Learning to recognise that feelings of guilt and shame are undeserved, can lead to deeper healing of trauma.

It is not your fault that you were abused, and there is nothing for you to feel guilty and ashamed about. It is the perpetrator who should feel guilty and ashamed.

When thoughts or feelings of guilt or shame come up, try to challenge them and remind yourself that you have done nothing wrong.

Guilt in sexual relationships

Sexual abuse can often affect intimate relationships. It is very common for survivors to feel guilty about wanting or engaging in consensual sex following an experience of sexual abuse, no matter how long ago it occurred.

You may have had thoughts such as "if I am able to have sex, I should be over it", "if I enjoy sex, people won't believe I was raped" or "it's bad of me to want something that has hurt me in the past".

Many survivors of sexual abuse and rape have felt like this. However, it is important to challenge these thoughts and feelings. You have just as much right to a healthy sex life as anyone else.

Learning to separate rape or sexual abuse from sex is an important part of healing. Healthy sex is entirely different from the violation involved in rape and sexual violence, even if the physical acts are the same.

Real life stories 7

A client told me that she has never told anyone and felt disgusted with her self, with what she had done. One therapy session, when it got the better of her, as we talked about, things that happen in life and talking about them, most of the time made it better for the person rather than keeping inside of them.

She told me that she was 17 and had gone into the woods with her cousin who was 18 and they had sex, just once. They both wanted to have sex.

They both knew that it would be seen as incest. She was so relieved to have told someone and not to have been judged by her actions.

No action was taken.

About the exercise:

This exercise is designed to help you identify and let go of some of the feelings of guilt and shame. Remember that whatever you are feeling, however strange, distressing or shameful it may feel to you, it is a completely normal reaction to an extreme and difficult situation.

You are not alone in feeling this way or having these thoughts.

How to complete this exercise:

Write down any thoughts and feelings relating to the questions labelled A. Once you have read them back, write next to them a challenge to that thought, an argument against the feelings, next to question B. You can use the example below to help you.

For example:

A) Is there anything about your experience of sexual abuse that makes you feel guilty?

I feel guilty when I think about how much it will upset my partner when I tell him.

B) How can you challenge this thought or feeling?

It is not my fault I was raped. The guilt is not mine to bear.

Real life stories 8

I always thought it normal that my father would touch me a lot when he was bathing me at night times, he always seem so close to me, I was 6 years old at the time and this went on till I was 12.

Only then did I realise what he had been doing to me.

I will never forgive him.

Now you try.

A) Is there anything about your experience of sexual abuse or rape that makes you feel guilty?

B) How can you challenge this thought or feeling?

A) Is there anything about your experience of sexual abuse or rape that makes you feel ashamed?

B) How can you challenge this thought or feeling?

Real life stories 9

I worked with a gentleman, who used to enjoy hanging outside a young girls school at lunchtime, the girls were aged 9 – 14 at this school.

He would place a white sheet by the school gates so that the girls would have to all walk over it as they went to lunch break.

He then would pick it up and take it home and masturbate with it. Now on the sex register list after serving 15 years in prison.

Section Five: Removing the Movie

Coping with flashbacks and intrusive thoughts

Flashbacks, intrusive thoughts and nightmares are very common in survivors of sexual abuse. They occur because, in a bid to protect itself, the mind shuts off the traumatic memories to make the distressing experience easier to process.

A side effect of this 'shutting off' however is that the memories and difficult emotions erupt elsewhere, through flashbacks, nightmares or intrusive thoughts.

They can cause anxiety and distress, but it is possible to work through these memories to get to a point where you can deal with them effectively.

About the exercise:

This is an exercise which can be used to alleviate some of the suffering associated with traumatic events in people lives. This exercise can be very successful in removing some of the distressing emotions associated with traumatic memories.

The process of this exercise is based on the principles of Neuro-Linguistic Programming. It involves replaying the visual memory of the experience of sexual violence. This method disrupts the painful way fears are remembered and enables the person's mind to re-code the traumatic event in a way that is less distressing.

Real life stories 10

I was working with a client on a confidence building exercise and half way through she just happen to mention that she had been date raped 2 weeks ago. This changed the whole exercise, as you can imagine.

She then quickly said the classic line "I deserved it" "I'm sorry" I said, why did you say that. "I sleep around a bit" she replied. To which I replied "I don't care if you sleep around or not, it doesn't justify you being date raped".

She took no action about the man that had raped her.

How to complete the exercise:

Find a comfortable place to sit down where you will not be disturbed for about twenty minutes. Please read through the steps and then do the exercise.

Now close your eyes and relax. Picture in your mind the inside of your favorite movie theater. Glance around the theater and notice that you have the whole place to yourself. You are safe. Visualize the colour of the walls, and what colour the seats are like.

See the large screen up front of you, the rows of empty comfortable chairs, and the exit signs.

Look back behind you and up for a moment to where the projection booth window is up on the rear wall, the box that the light comes out of.

Now find the best seat in the theater, and settle into it. Take in the sights, sounds and smells of the theater. Feel the seat and floor underneath you.

Now look up on the movie screen you can see a black and white still photo of yourself. It's just a BORING picture, such as you washing up, hanging the washing out, or a child playing with a familiar toy or sitting on the sofa. It's just a single picture of you, taken before you had the traumatic experience, which the movie is going to play in a few minutes. If you can't think of a photo, just make one up, it will work just as well.

Soon, the screen is going to show a black and white movie about you. This movie will have no sound, it will play like a poor quality home video, and it may even flicker a bit.

Now that you are comfortable in the seat, watching the still black and white picture of yourself, before the movie starts, let your "body" drift up behind you into the projection booth where you can control the movie, while the physical "you" person remains relaxed in the theater seat.

Float your body up to the projection booth now.

Look around the booth, and note the details of the walls and each side of you the exit. Notice the frame around the window, and the large reels of film on the projector, and see the long beam of dusty white light streaming towards the movie screen. As you look out of the small glass window, you notice how thick the glass is, you are very safe and feel protected.

Look down through the glass window and see you sitting in your favorite seat watching the screen, waiting for the movie to start.

In a moment the movie will start in black and white, it will start from a time when you are safe and didn't know the traumatic event was going to happen, and the movie will end after you are back in a safe place after the event.

So now looking through the little glass window, see yourself down in the theater seat, and as you look up to the screen, the movie starts. Watch the scratchy black-and-white movie, of you going through your traumatic experience, as it begins to play on the screen.

The movie starts at a time shortly before the event and plays on through the event and then continues on to a time well after the event, when you are in a safe and protected space. Then the movie ends. The screen goes blank.

Now, float yourself from the projection booth down into the seat where you're sitting, see yourself stand up and walk down the isle and go up on stage to the movie screen.

See the end of the movie scene now through your own eyes. Notice that the movie now becomes fully dimensional – with full colour and sound. Step into the movie and become yourself at the end of the movie.

In a minute, quickly play the film backwards, this time in colour. The people move backwards, add a soundtrack of a silly tune that makes you laugh, with you in the movie. Now, Step into and become you in the movie. Rewind it all the way back to the beginning. Do this very fast in 5 seconds. The screen goes blank. Do it now.

Now you're back in the projection booth, float yourself from the projection booth down into the seat where your sitting, see yourself stand up and walk down the aisle and go up on stage to the movie screen. Enter the movie at the end again.

Now quickly, play the film backwards, this time in colour. The people move backwards, the sound of the silly tune that makes you laugh, with you in the movie, also moving backwards. Rewind it all the way back to the beginning. Do this even faster in 3 seconds this time. Go.

Now you're back in the projection booth, float yourself from the projection booth down into the seat where you're sitting, see yourself stand up and walk down the aisle and go up on stage to the movie screen.

Now quickly, play the film backwards, this time in colour. The people move backwards, the sound of a silly tune that makes you laugh, with you in the movie, also moving backwards. Rewind it all the way back to the beginning. Do this so fast the whole experience is done in 1 second from end to the beginning. Go.

Now, think of a time you enjoyed strawberries or another lovely fruit you enjoy, smell it, taste it and see it.

Explore how you feel about that situation now, and maybe how differently now you start to feel.

Stop the exercise here, if things have changed for you in your mind.

Remember you are not looking to get total removal, just changing your experience of the memory, which will enable you to move forward now.

Now, if you feel it would be helpful, you can play the movie backwards again.

But this time, allow yourself to listen to a different tune maybe the funniest, most ludicrous background music you can imagine, something from a circus act or a disco nightclub, maybe.

Now you're back in the projection booth, float yourself from the projection booth down into the seat where you're sitting, see yourself stand up and walk down the isle and go up on stage to the movie screen.

Now quickly, play the film backwards, this time in colour. The people move backwards, the sound is of a silly tune that makes you laugh, with you in the movie, also moving backwards.

Rewind it all the way back to the beginning.

Do this again 3 times as before, taking only 5 seconds, then 3 seconds and finally just 1 second.

Real life stories 11

A yoga teacher came for a therapy session one day for confidence building, half away through the session, she started talking about her relationship with her new husband and that they were trying for a chid, who she loves.

She said that they had an argument one night recently and she went out and got drunk, she went home with another man that night and that she had got pregnant.

She didn't know what to do. She never told her husband and they now have a lovely son.

Section Six: Time to Relax

Why is relaxation important?

Following experiences of sexual abuse or rape, the effects of trauma and emotions such as fear and anger may be seen in mental, emotional and physical health.

This may be true whether the traumatic event happened recently, or a long time ago. In addition, coping with secrecy or worrying about things that might happen in the future can cause a lot of stress hormones to be released which can be damaging to the immune system and organ function.

Relaxation exercises can help to promote more feelings of calm and balance, while reducing the amount of stress hormones released.

Learning ways to cope with difficult emotions can therefore help to improve our emotional and physical health.

About the exercise:

This exercise, named 'The Rainbow Garden' is part of a holistic approach to caring for mind, body and spirit during recovery from trauma. In this exercise you will practice deep self communication.

You will use relaxation and imagery to stimulate your imagination. By increasing your self awareness, you can learn to heal, balance, and center yourself.

This exercise uses colour psychology to unlock different benefits associated with different colours:

- RED stimulates the five senses, builds the liver and blood and cleanses and purifies the skin.

- ORANGE supports the lungs, thyroid, and bones. Relieves cramps and muscle spasms.

- YELLOW stimulates the lymph system, intestines, pancreas, and balances out melancholy.

- GREEN stimulates and balances the pituitary, stimulates building of muscle tissue, destroys germs and prevents decay.

- VIOLET builds the spleen, tranquilizes the nervous system, decreases sensitivity to pain and allows the heart muscle to work less.

- BLUE stimulates the pineal gland, builds vitality, removes fever, and is a mild sedative.

- WHITE holds all the other colours within it and motivates us as a balanced unit to function in a loving, peaceful and positive mode.

How to complete the exercise:

Sit or lie comfortably. Take three deep breaths and relax.

You could record this exercise yourself or maybe get someone to read this section to you.

So now, begin to visualize yourself near a beautiful hillside that stretches gently upward in front of you. Find yourself at the foot of this gentle hill just following a spring shower and see a beautiful rainbow of many colours stretching up over a hill and coming to rest just in front of you. At the end of the rainbow that comes to just in front of you, see a beautiful pouch.

Pick up this pouch and look inside and see there are many magical seeds. Magical seeds that you can scatter on your way. And now begin to walk forward to the bottom of the hill. Reach inside your pouch and scatter some of the magical seeds. In just a moment, see these magical seeds begin to grow and bloom. See a profusion of red blooming flowers. See the bright red poppies growing near the ground. Smell the rich odor of red roses nearby.

See red tulips opening to the morning sun. Experience the feeling of red all around you. And as you walk forward through the deep red flowers, appreciate your own physical nature. Remember the physical sensations which bring you comfort and pleasure. Appreciate all of your physical senses, which allow you to be part of life and to experience the fullness and joy of living.

Continue to walk upward along the gentle slope of your hill, reaching again into your pouch and scatter more seeds. Feel the sense of expectancy for a new birth of orange blossoms, bursting into bloom around you. Cast your eyes on the field of orange surrounding you. See tufts of orange marigolds. Watch the birth of crocuses, orange buds opening to the light. See birds of paradise growing profusely and filling your awareness with the colour orange.

Visualize an increased growth of the colour orange. Reflect for a moment on the value of contact with your fellow human beings. Appreciate the importance of interaction with others. Realize that you gain through social activities and contact with other people. Recognize the beautiful ability you have to interact with fellow human beings.

Now allow yourself to move into the next region of the chakra garden. Feel your awareness glow with anticipation as you scatter your magic seeds.

Experience the strong bold essence of yellow. See sunflowers growing strong and tall yellow light reflected from their petals. Pass through the daffodils and feel their yellow cups caressing you. Walk gently forward and experience and appreciate the beauty and fragrance of the yellow roses. See their delicate petals unfolding before your eyes. Scatter your seeds with assurance that the growth of yellow will flourish.

For the moment appreciate your ability to be discriminating – to flow with change and to make decisions which will make your life and those around you have more meaning. Relax and flow with the feeling of gratitude for change, knowing that change for a soul walking towards the light always denotes growth. Know that through change real growth can take place.

Begin to move upward where you reach the next region of the hillside garden. Reach into your pouch again and with your magical seeds you feel a deep sense of inner peace as you scatter seeds which bring forth a lush green growth. See new grasses and new clover springing up around you. Experience the fresh scent of green pine needles. See the tiny green leaves of aspen trees fluttering beyond number and sounding like spring rain in the gentle breeze.

As you scatter your seeds which promise a continuing expansion of green, feel the security of the presence of life and light deep within you. Get in touch with the health of your body. Feel strength grow deep within you. Know that you are in control of your health.

Continue to travel onward to the next region of your grassy knoll and scatter your magic seeds with a marvellous appreciation for the bluebells springing up to greet you as you walk.

Feel yourself saturated with the feeling of blue blossoms. Look around at the bushes of lilacs and take another handful of seeds and scatter them, growing blue flowers. Anticipate the lush growth of blue. Take a moment and revel at your ability to take a look inside yourself.

Feel yourself stopping by a pool of water where irises grow in lush abundance. Look into the water and see the hue of the irises brilliantly reflected. Take a drink from this fresh stream.

Be grateful for your ability to know that this is the energy and nature of your true being which you allow to be expressed every day in love, peace and harmony.

When you close your eyes for sleep, this is also the beautiful, peaceful place you go for renewing, restoring and revitalizing your being. Assure yourself now that every day in your awareness of this beautiful blue energy you trust intuition and knowledge to magnify more and more.

In continuing your upward path you reach inside your pouch spreading more seeds to find yourself in a vast expanse which surrounds your feet and legs in a lovely field of violets. Feel yourself experiencing lavender and violet and let the colour permeate your being.

Gaze and let your eyes fill with this color of the uppermost part of the garden. Cast the seeds which will allow an endless growth of violet. Appreciate your ability to create powerful images and to be totally in charge of your life.

From this region of the garden, look to the sky and see the pure light of the sun, visualize rays of sunshine showering the entire garden and feel ripples of vibration as drops of pure brilliant light shower the garden with loving energy.

Move upward to the very top of the hill and scatter the remaining seeds around you. Now see and feel a beautiful profusion of white roses growing close to you.

Feel a great joy in the knowledge that every one of the colours and essences you have experienced in The Rainbow Garden are a necessary part of your being and in experiencing the colours and forms you identify with the oneness of all life energy.

All aspects of your being vibrate on the various colours, energy frequencies and all are open to your demand and control for change.

All of life's colours and energies needs are open to your recognition and appreciation. Bringing a new awareness of life's beauty, and life's love that surrounds you.

As you begin to walk back down life's hillside, through the violet, the blue, the green, the yellow, the orange and the red flowers, know that you can return to this hillside garden any time you wish and that each time you do return your inner being and your outer being will have a new awareness of the hillside.

As you grow and develop in all aspects of your being, the world around you will change and beauty will surround you.

The Rainbow Garden CD is available from the website

www.mysilenceisbroken.com

Section Seven –
Deciding Who to Tell or 'If' to Tell

Deciding if, and who, to tell about your experience of sexual abuse or rape can be a very difficult process. This may be for many reasons.

Sometimes the person who has abused you will make you feel that nobody will believe you and that nobody cares about what is happening to you. This is simply not true, and is a way that abusers try to prevent repercussions for them.

If the abuse happened a long time ago, you may feel that it is not worth telling anyone about what happened. If your abuser was a member of your family, friend group, work environment or community, you may feel scared to speak out about your experience in case it causes problems.

Talking about and gaining support in dealing with sexual abuse can be one of the major stepping stones in moving on with your life. You may feel scared to do so, worried about what others will think, or that you will not be believed. You may be scared to say because it might disrupt a settled environment

Remember that you have nothing to be ashamed about. It is not your fault. The only person who should feel ashamed and worried about what others will think should be the perpetrator.

Choosing the right person to talk to about your experience and feelings is very important. It should be someone you feel safe with, who you can trust to keep your confidence, and who will not pressure you to make decisions. The person you choose to tell should be able to help you:

- To feel understood and supported
- To feel listened to
- To feel that you are believed
- To be supported to access help _when_ you ask for it
- To be supported if going to the police station
- To feel that they understand that your life in may be very different from now on

The person you choose to tell should not:

- Tell you what to do, e.g. go to the police
- Take control of the situation
- Direct abuse towards the perpetrator or seek revenge
- Keep asking what happened
- Ask why you didn't tell someone
- Tell you that you will be ok after a few weeks, or that it will pass
- Blame you in any way, such as asking why you did not struggle, or if you led the person on.

About the exercise:

This exercise is designed to help you think about the right person for you, to be able to feel safe and supported while speaking about your experience.

There is no pressure to immediately tell anyone, but going through this exercise may help you to feel that there is support around you if and when you do decide to speak out.

"If and when you tell someone, this is a very positive step. You are beginning to trust someone again".

How to complete the exercise:

Complete the following sentences and or choose from the options available.

Who is in your support circle? Tick any of the people you currently have around you who you trust and feel safe with.

Partner

Close friends

Mother

Father

Sister

Brother

Child

Cousin

Other family member

Doctor or nurse

Counsellor or therapist

Member of your religious community

Teacher

Colleague

Police officer

Support worker

Social worker

Other

Choose between one and three people from the list which you ticked. What do you think they would say if you told them? Refer back to the lists of what a supportive person should and shouldn't do.

1) One person I could trust to support me is:

I think they would say:

I would feel safe speaking to them because:

2) A second person I could trust to support me is:

I think they would say:

I would feel safe speaking to them because:

3) A third person I could trust to support me is:

I think they would say:

I would feel safe speaking to them because:

Section Eight – The Future You

Who is the future you?

Now that you are becoming more empowered and taking steps to move on with your life, it is good to think about what the future you is like.

Sexual abuse and rape can take us to the darkest places in our minds.

The trauma can have a huge effect on the way we behave, feel and perceive the world.

However, the work that you are doing has been proven to help with moving forward and building a life that you love.

Survivors of sexual abuse do heal, recover, move forward, build great relationships and get their life back. You will, too.

"Remember, you can't reach what's in front of you until you let go of what's behind you"

~ Chinna Sharma

About the exercise:

This exercise asks you to write some thoughts and feelings about your plans and dreams for the future, the relationships you want to develop and the way you want to live your life. This is just a start to new beginnings for you.

How to complete the exercise

Complete the following questions, using extra paper as needed.

Enjoyment of Life

What activities or experiences in your life at the moment do you really enjoy?

What would you like to do more of?

What new things, whether hobbies, interests, career aspirations or travel plans, would you like to try in the future?

What are you looking forward to?

Relationships

What are you looking for in a relationship?

If you are in a current relationship, has anything changed in the relationship? How do you feel about it?

What support would you like and what understanding would you like to receive in your relationship?

Feeling Supported

How are you feeling now, after all the great work you have done in this work book?

Has there been a change since the beginning of the process?

Is there other support that you would like to receive, that you are currently not getting at present?

Take a moment now to congratulate yourself on getting this far. You have taken some brave first steps into healing and moving on.

Show yourself some love and appreciation for the courage you have shown.

This coupon entitles the owner to

ONE FREE HUG

Redeemable anytime

Then give 10 of these to someone who is very supportive of you.

Remember to redeem your loving HUGS

Section Nine - Some Suggested Reading

This is a small selection of books available on the themes of healing from sexual abuse and rape; there are plenty more available as well.

MY FATHER'S HOUSE

A Memoir of the incest and of Healing

Sylvia Fraser – ISBN: 080606 81815

THE OBSIDIAN MIRROR

An Adult Healing from Incest

Louise Wisechild – ISBN: 18780 67397

SHINING THROUGH

Pulling it Together after Sexual Abuse

Mindy B Loiselle and Leslie Bailey Wright - ISBN:18844 4413X

THE SURVIVORS GUIDE

Sharice A. Lee – ISBN: 08039 57815

TOP SECRET
Sexual Assault information for Teenagers Only
Jennifer Fay & Billie Jo Flerchinger – ISBN: 09419 53106

RESCUING THE "INNER CHILD"
Therapy for Adults – Sexually Abused Children
Penny Parks – ISBN: 02856 50890

STRONG AT THE BROKEN PLACES
Overcoming the Trauma of Childhood Abuse
Linda Sanford – ISBN: 18538 13745

Thank you for your time working through this workbook.

Please remember, you are not alone and it was not your fault.

www.mysilenceisbroken.com

Further information and training available:

www.mysilenceisbroken.com

1-2-1 support available / Phone / Email / Skype

Co-Founder of Healing Connections Magazine. Now in its 10th year with a print of over 9000 copies and comes out 3 times a year. www.healingconnectionsmagazine.com

Business NLP Training / Coaching / Hypnotherapy / Counselling / CBT / Mindfulness

Past clients include: Harrods, Elstree Film Studios, Heals, House of Fraser, Marks and Spencer, Freedom Communications, John Lewis and many more.

Sports Coaching / Personal Training – Has worked with top UK Athletes who then went on to win British and European gold medals.

Currently part of the Medical Team and Pitch side Medic at Wembley Stadium. Experience of working at the Champions League Final 2013, The Olympics 2012 and the Rugby World Cup Final 2015.

Enjoyed working with the YMCA Central London. As a Positive Health Instructor. Working with HIV and AIDS groups for just under 2 years.

Licence for the Gastric Hypno-Band - Weight Loss System

Animal Healing / Animal Behaviour training

Ran talks and workshops in Richmond South Virginia. USA

Published in ES magazine and Kindred Spirit Magazine in the UK

Various Hypnotherapy CD's / MP3's available.

Second book now available –

Weight Loss – The Thin book for Thin people

Both books are available on Amazon worldwide and Kindle format

- Future books to look out for:

- Animal healing – Understanding your animals
- Naturally Feminine – Reshaping your body through the power of your mind
- Colour Your Body
- Improving your eyesight naturally

Gary Sellors can be contacted on:
- wellbeingconsultant@hotmail.co.uk
- LinkedIn
- www.garysellors.com